MORNING BLESSINGS

By Veronica Gordon

With Ruth C. Chapman

V

MORNING

BLESSINGS

BY VERONICA GORDON

WITH RUTH C. CHAPMAN

V

"Who shall find a virtuous woman?
For her price is far above rubies. The
heart of her husband doth safely trust
in her. Her children rise up and call her
blessed."

Proverbs 31:10

Veronica Gordon and her husband, Delroy have been instrumental in implementing a dynamic health reform movement in Puerto, Viejo, Costa Rica. Together with their five children, they have established a successful ministry of healthy holistic living.

DEDICATION

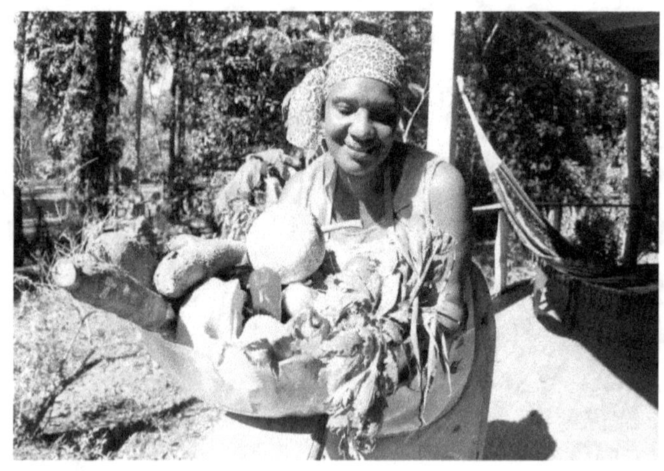

This book is dedicated to all who rise early to seek the wonders of God and to dwell in His presence in the start of the day.

FOREWORD

It is in the early morning hours that God feels most present to me. It is in that time that my mind, body, spirit and soul awaken with Him. I thank Him. I praise Him. I glorify Him. For most of my life I have awakened early to dwell in God's presence before I would begin to face the rigors of the day. It was always in my quiet time alone with God that I could fellowship with Him alone. "What a fellowship! What a joy divine!" To me, there is no splendor that can compare with quiet time alone with God.

Last year, while visiting family in Costa Rica, I discovered a new layer of fellowship with God. I found the fellowship with God joined by the fellowship of a dear friend. Walking along the beach, praying, meditating, sharing testimonies and resting to observe the beauty of God's creation were the morning blessings of early morning fellowship with a friend.

Several times a week during my stay in Costa Rica, I would meet with my dear sister/friend Veronica Gordon. We would begin our walks during sunrise, just chatting along the way to the ocean. When we would reach a quiet alcove under the shade of a Noni tree, we would rest on a dry, but sandy log by the ocean's edge and pray. It was with our prayer that God would infuse Veronica with the wisdom He desired for us for this day. "Give us this day, our daily bread." Prayer was like bread for our souls. After we set our minds on Him for guidance, Veronica would rely on God to give her the thoughts she wanted to include in this book. I would rely on God to give me the ability to hear with a spiritual ear, so I could "write the words and make them plain." We continued our walk surrounded by the magnificence of God's handiwork. By the end of our walk, we were both filled with the joy of spending time with God in the early part of the day.

These pages are the result of the wisdom God poured into Veronica. I feel enormously blessed to have been able to be a part of these daily MORNING BLESSINGS.

With Great Appreciation to God and my dear Sister/Friend Veronica Gordon.

Love and Blessings,

Ruth C. Chapman

INTRODUCTION

MORNING BLESSINGS

"Give us this day our daily bread."

Getting our minds ready for the day starts when we wake up. If we want to get our minds ready in the physical, we must be conducted by the Holy Spirit. We should begin our day by serving God for that day. We must focus on serving God and living our lives one day at a time. When God directed his people in the wilderness, He directed them to pick up only what they would need for that day for them and their family. The same is true of our spiritual life that is guided by the Holy Spirit.

"Morning by morning, new mercies I see."

God wants us to begin thinking on the things we desire to do on that day, and how

V

we should serve Him. As it is with food, we must try to take in spiritual nourishment, chew it properly, and assimilate it for our spiritual sustenance.

Each day we get new nourishment for our mind, body and spirit. God wants us to be responsible for managing what He has given. The Holy Spirit is our source of spiritual nourishment from God. We must focus on our daily bread. Every day, we must rely on the power of the Holy Spirit to give us what we need for our daily nourishment.

HUMILITY AND HUMANITY

Our spiritual provisions are not to be used selfishly or for vainglory. We are to reach out to mankind with humility after we have received of Him.

V

A PERSONAL PRAYER

"LORD, I ASK YOU TO TRANSFORM ME BEFORE I START MY DAY. PUT YOUR SPIRIT IN ME TO SERVE OTHERS AND THE ABILITY TO RELY ON YOU BEFORE I REACH OUT TO OTHERS. GIVE ME A HEART OF FLESH AND TAKE AWAY MY STONY HEART. HELP ME TO LISTEN AS YOU SPEAK TO ME. GIVE ME MY INSTRUCTIONS. FILL ME WITH WHAT I NEED TO SERVE YOU TODAY. AMEN"

GOD BLESS YOU!

Veronica Gordon

V

Thankfulness

"Thank you for waking me this morning.

Thank you for giving me today.

Thank you for every bright tomorrow.

Thanks for everything."

(Words to a morning song of praise sung by Veronica Gordon)

MORNING

BLESSINGS

BY VERONICA GORDON

WITH RUTH C. CHAPMAN

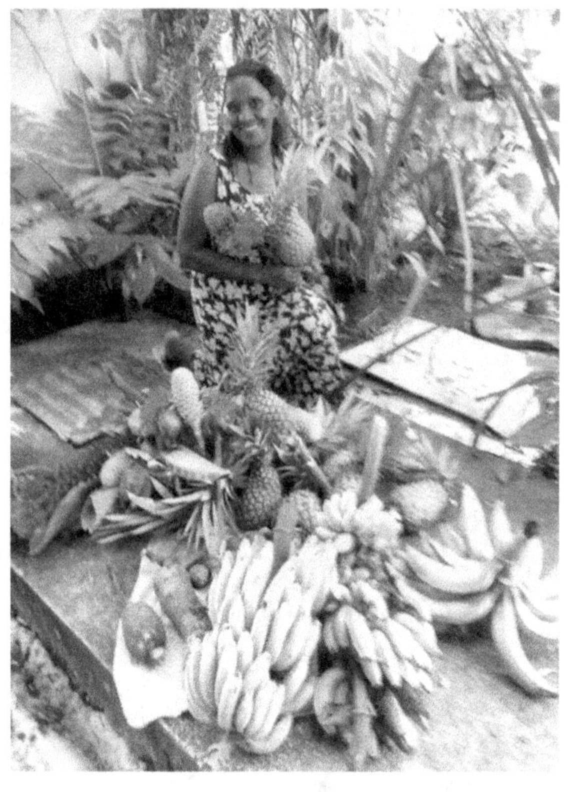

"I will bless the Lord at all times. His praise shall continually be in my mouth. My soul shall make her boast in the Lord...Oh magnify the Lord with me! Let us exalt His name together!"

Psalm 34:1

BREATH

"The Lord God formed the man from the dust of the earth and breathed into his nostrils the breath of life, and man became a living soul." Genesis 2:7

BREATH/AIR

The living soul must be taken care of through our dedication to God. We are an integrated being of mind, body and spirit. God will guide us on how to take care of ourselves.

The bible prepares us and teaches us about who God is and how He works. He wants us to regard our body as the temple of the Holy Spirit. We must take care of our temple to preserve it for service and protect it from destruction. We must respect the body which is powered by the breath of life.

FOOD

What we eat is what we are. We must follow God's guidance. Our bodies will not live forever, but through proper nourishment and attentive maintenance, we can help our bodies to live with more health, strength, and vitality. Life offers many alternatives and food options. It is our responsibility to make the best choices for a happy and healthy life that is fulfilling and productive.

We should find the lessons in God's Word. This body must be taken care of and protected. The destruction of the body, due to poor nourishment is a process. It does not happen suddenly. It happens in phases until the body is no longer healthy.

Our bodies were designed to work in sync with nature. Nature was designed to heal our bodies. The five senses help us to be aware of what is good and what is harmful. We must be in tune with God's guidance. Pay attention to what we see, hear, touch, smell and taste. If something does not agree with your bodies, you should exclude it from our diets and our lifestyles. God gives us free choice. We are not robots. God made us in His image to live according to His will. We must be careful to not allow our will to override God's will. God's will is for us to live a life with health, joy and vigor. It is not God's desire that we live long unhealthy and unhappy lives.

"...LIVE THIS LIFE AND THAT MORE ABUNDANTLY."

Nourishing our bodies properly opens our brains to hear God's will and follow His plan for an abundant life. The body is consistently weakened by poor dietary practices. Today, there are a lot of diseases that are prevalent because of the way foods are processed. Our bodies do not know how to process synthetic, artificial foods. Pure and natural foods contain all the vitamins, minerals and nutrients that our bodies need. The brain needs to be clear to make the best choices for health, wellness and living in general.

Take time in the morning to give your body the nourishment it needs. That would help give you what we need to combat disease and strengthen and heal our bodies. The less we use synthetics, artificial colors, or preservatives in our food, the more we give our bodies the opportunity to have a good start and maintain balance.

V

PROPER ELIMINATION

Equally important as putting into our bodies the things that are pure and wholesome, is eliminating from our bodies the things that are harmful. Fiber is necessary to help the body function properly and eliminate what the body does not need. Include fiber that is also filled with proteins, minerals and vitamins. To assure that you have ample amounts of fiber available in your home, food planning is vital. By planning properly, you are more likely to eat what is wholesome instead of grabbing unhealthy substitutes because of mere convenience. In planning, food portions should be considered as well. When you are more attentive to what you are eating, and the benefits of your chosen diets, you will be more likely to be mindful of eating healthy amounts. Preparing foods ahead of time and storing them in proper amounts to be eaten in single servings helps deter you from over-indulging. Your body will determine for you what portions are appropriate for your body. Some people skimp on meals and deprive the body of what it needs for energy and nutrition. Eat plentiful amounts of nutritious foods and stop eating when you begin to feel full and satisfied. It is tempting to eat too little or too much simply because of what we desire. Foods that are high in sugar, fats, starches and artificial ingredients may taste good, and have you wanting more, but in the long run, these foods are not giving your body what it needs. On the other hand, some people over-indulge based on false messages. Seeing or smelling something that you like can trick you into thinking you want more. That is something that advertisers know very well. Do not let yourself be lulled into thinking that you need something because it is there in front of you.

Monitor your portions and eat what your body needs. When your body says stop eating, listen to what it is telling you. God helps you to know what is right and good for you.

We have gotten away from healthy practices. It is important to modify what we do and train ourselves to listen to our bodies. There are natural signals that tell us what is good for us. It is important to listen to our bodies and heed the natural messages given.

"...Whatsoever things are true, whatsoever things are honest, whatsoever things are pure, whatsoever things are lovely, whatsoever things are of good report; if there be any virtue, and if there be any praise, think on these things."

Philippians 4:8

MENTAL PREPAREDNESS

Plan each day to begin with a focus on positive thoughts. There is always something for which to be grateful. To be able to use your mind with clear thought is a blessing. To be able to use your senses is a blessing. The ability to have the use of your body with relative ease is a source of joy.

Share your joy and your blessings to give God and others a joyful heart. When we give God thanks and praise, He delights in us. When we share our joy with others, it helps lift burdens and gives encouragement. Think of ways at the start of the day to praise God and bless others throughout the day.

The patterns in nature give us a pattern to use to start the day. Tune into the patterns provided by nature and train your mind to follow those examples.

PHYSICAL PRESERVATION

Start with Water

The moment we drink water, hydration begins. Water hydrates every portion of our body, including the brain. Drinking water early in the morning helps the brain to focus more clearly to start the day properly and carry out our daily tasks more effectively.

Remember that water is essential. Drink water first thing in the morning. Water flushes our bodies of impurities. Water keeps our bodies, especially our digestive systems, regulated. We should be able to urinate numerous times in a day. By drinking eight glasses of water a day, we should be able to urinate a clear stream every few

V

hours. We should be able to eliminate waste from our bowels at least 3 times a day. The more food we have in the bowel track without eliminating regularly keeps poisons in the system. Poisons produce disease. One disease that is on the rise is colon cancer. You can help deter the buildup of poisons by flushing impurities out of your colon and other parts of your system.

Eliminating first thing in the morning gives your system a clean start for the day. Once the body has eliminated the waste materials, your body is ready to receive the nutrients that can be absorbed and utilized for health and healing.

What we put in our bodies at the start of our day, helps keep us sustained throughout the day. Therefore, cleanse your body with a refreshing flow of water. Our bodies are comprised mostly of water. Keeping our bodies in balance with the proper amount of water is essential.

Drinking the amount of water necessary helps our brain to wake up. Water helps our digestive system to cleanse itself. As a child, my elders said that we must drink water and be willing to offer water to those who lack it. Offering a cool drink of water is a hospitable gesture. It is a sign of offering a blessing upon a person. The blessing of water helps us spiritually, emotionally, physically, and socially. Water is a blessing and we should pray and thank God for the blessings that He so plentifully provides for us.

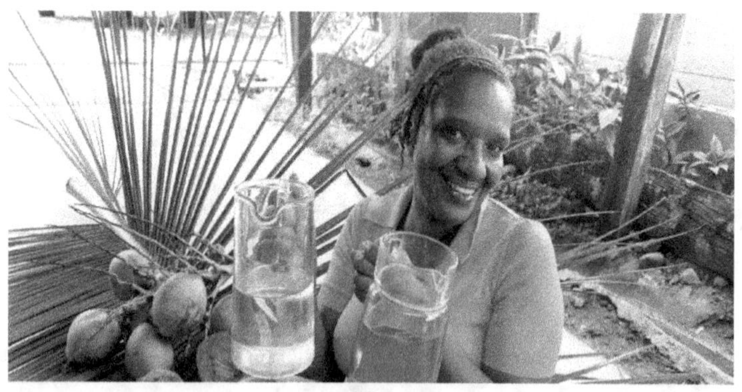

Follow with Fruit

Fruit contains a large portion of water. Eating fruit provides nourishment and hydration. Eat the fruit you enjoy either singularly or in a healthy fruit salad. About one half hour after drinking your morning portion of water, follow with a generous serving of fruit. This will give your body the boost it needs to continue the process of nourishing and hydrating the body. Fruit contains vitamins, minerals, and a good amount of fiber. Although most fruits do contain natural sugar, it is easily absorbed into the body. You can begin to feel full by eating a substantial amount of fruit without great concerns about consuming more calories than the body needs. Some people desire a cup of natural herbal tea after their serving of fruit. There are many choices of natural teas made from plants that help the body with healing and health. Including lime with your morning tea helps provide the alkaline balance that your body needs. Drinking warm herbal tea unsweetened is preferred, but if you desire, add a small amount of natural honey to sweeten your drink.

Now that you have given your body ample water and sufficient amounts of fruits, you are now ready for the main portion of your meal to begin your day.

SOLID FOODS SUSTAIN

Finish your morning meal with more solid foods to give sustenance for the day. Food is your energy source. Eat enough to feel satisfied with a good solid amount of nourishment. A good breakfast should sustain you for up to four hours. So, eat enough to fill you, but not to make you uncomfortable or sluggish. Be mindful that if you have eaten sufficiently, you should not feel hungry until it is time for your next meal. Often, people mistake thirst for hunger. If you are feeling hungry, try drinking water. It may be what your body is craving. When drinking water to stave off hunger, remember to refrain from drinking water for at least one half an hour before your next meal. Drinking water too soon before a meal or even during a meal interferes with proper digestion.

Our food needs to be integral or wholesome. Foods that are refined and filled with additives do not provide us with the right nutrients. Our bodies do not feel full or satisfied with foods that are not wholesome.

Eat enough in the morning to keep you energized. If you do physical work, you need a more substantial breakfast. If you are more sedentary, you can eat less. Find the proper amount for you personally.

Now that you have given your body the great start that it needs, you are ready to face the day!

HAVE A GOOD DAY! ENJOY!

V

"We are fearfully and wonderfully made."

The first thing in the morning, even before we arise from our beds, we can begin to exercise our bodies. We can begin with the most modest movements. We can begin by simply opening our eyes and stretching them wide. Look to each side and up and down. Continue by looking around at our surroundings. What goes through our eyes, goes right to our brain. This would be a good time to give God thanks for the gift of sight, the ability to move your eyes freely, and for the provisions He has made. We can follow that with a wide yawn and a large stretch. Yawning forces oxygen into our brains and lungs. Our entire blood system relies on oxygen to function properly. Stretching and sending oxygen through our bodies allows our muscles to become more relaxed and better able to support our skeletal system and prevent injury. If you observe nature, you will notice that most of God's creatures move their bodies slowly and deliberately before moving into action. Sudden movements can cause pain and injury. Bodies need to warm up before becoming engaged with the demands of the day.

"For in Him we live and move and have our being." Acts 17:28

V

STRETCHING

By stretching our bodies, we are also stretching our mind and our spirit. Everything that moves is praising God. Use this time of stretching to praise God. Be attentive to the ways in which your body can stretch. Every muscle, every bone, every sinew, tendon and ligament work together to be stronger and longer. The more we stretch, the further we can stretch. Stretching helps eliminate pain. Muscles and joints may be stiff in the morning. So, stretch them out to reduce the aches throughout the day. Be gentle. Joints and muscles need time to warm up and get fluid flowing. Not only do muscles and joints need fluids to flow, but also, the brain needs adequate blood flow to help you think clearly and to concentrate. Stretching in the morning is a great way to get energy throughout your body from head to toe.

Take note of gradual improvements over time and thank God for the growth He gives.

Water and stretching work together to enable the brain flow to send blood and nutrients to the right places in the body to help the body to be flexible.

A GRACEFUL, GRATEFUL ROUTINE

When you get out of bed, move around slowly to awaken your body. Go about the regular morning movements with a spirit of thankfulness and praise. Walk around the bedroom. Look out the window to take in the beauty of God's creation. Thank Him as you reflect on His goodness. Once you have taken time to reflect on God's goodness, proceed to the next steps of preparation for the day. Reach for the items you need for the day. Make your movements slow and deliberate so that you can stretch and subtly exercise your body. Shower or bathe with the purpose of cleansing the body and mentally washing away impurities. Even early in the day, it is tempting to have negative thoughts creep into your mind and spirit. Wash them away immediately and focus instead on those things that are pure, honest and lovely. Warm water relaxes the body, mind and spirit. As you allow your body to feel the healing sensation of water, tension disappears and calming, peaceful thoughts appear. As you gently and peacefully bathe, your circulation increases. Stress goes down the drain along with toxins. Taking time to shower or bathe in the morning produces a healthier, more radiant you, inside and out.

Water temperature is important to provide the purpose for which it is intended. Water temperature affects the body. Warm water is relaxing. It promotes rest and relaxation. A warm bath or shower at night helps the body to rest. Whereas, a cold or hot shower in the morning helps stimulate energy.

When you get dressed, do that with purpose as well. Thank God for providing clothing. and for allowing you to have the ability to dress yourself. Regardless of your age, occupation or ability level, dressing nicely and comfortably helps give an emotional boost. While it may not be necessary to get dressed up for your purpose, wearing nice, fresh, clean clothes is a plus. Clothing that permits the body to move comfortably helps you to remain comfortable throughout the day. Of course, it is important to protect your body with the clothes that are suitable for your environment. Depending on the climate in which you live, dress appropriately for the weather. If you live in a hot and humid climate, wearing cotton is a good idea. It is a breathable fabric that allows airflow and is good for absorption. If your climate is cold, heavier, natural fabrics are best.

Proper grooming is also a benefit to creating a sense of well-being. As far as grooming is concerned, you should always try to look and smell your best. There are many natural toiletries available that do an excellent job. Find or make grooming products that help you smell, look and feel fresh and clean. You will be blessed, and others will not be offended. There are so many things for which to be grateful. When you have done your morning routine with a grateful heart, your mind, body and spirit are all ready to move to the next level of exercise.

As mentioned previously, stretching is one of the easiest and most beneficial ways to awaken the body for the purposes of the day. Before moving on to a more demanding phase of exercise, stretch again. The arising stretching routine is primarily to ease your body into wakefulness. The next phase of stretching is to help your body to move with more vigor and vitality. After stretching gently and moving about with a purposeful, prayerful, meditative routine, you can begin a more focused exercise regimen as your schedule permits. Any amount of morning exercise can be helpful, but if your work schedule does not permit a full morning workout each day, arise early enough to ease into the day with the amount of exercise that is appropriate for you. Perhaps weekends or days that are less demanding may be excellent times to schedule a full workout routine. Each day do what you can.

THINK EIGHT

By focusing on the number 8, you can exercise several parts of your body. Start at the top with your head and neck and move downward until your reach your ankles and feet. With each part of your body, rotate in the motion of a figure 8:

Head and neck

Right arm

Left arm

Mid-section

Right leg

Left leg

Right foot

Left foot

Finally, shake your body gently to the count of eight. Do this as many times as you

V

wish. Now, your body is ready to keep going on to a more rigorous workout. Some people enjoy a fast- paced walk, while others prefer running. Swimming and biking are also excellent aerobic exercises.

Throughout the day, find ways to keep your body moving. If you observe children, they are in a state of almost perpetual motion. Try being more childlike in how you move your body. Better yet, when you have time, play with children and move as they move. Try skipping, jumping, hopping, playing sports and other games. Your children will cherish the time spent with them. You can develop a stronger less stressful bond. Whatever you do, do it with joy! Keep your heart pumping and filled with joy!

"A happy face makes the heart cheerful...."
Proverbs 15:13

(REST, REFLECT AND RENEW)

At the end of any vigorous exercise, allow your body to cool down and calm down. Take time to allow your body to gradually adjust. Ideally, you should move slowly, stretch gently and hydrate plentifully. Get your heartrate to ease its way to about 100 to 120 beats per minute. The health reform studies call for a lower number, but, in the United States, the above numbers are considered normal or desirable.

Walk slowly while reflecting on the blessings of God. If you have exercised with another person, this would be a good time to fellowship and perhaps share a testimony as you walk or sit to rest. The end of an exercise routine should leave you refreshed and renewed. Go forth with your day to share with others the manifold blessings that life has to offer!

V

"Then your light shall break forth like the morning. Your healing shall spring forth speedily."

Isaiah 58:8

"Where two or three are gathered together in my name, I am there in the midst."

Matthew 18:20

NOTE: Exercising for about a half an hour is adequate for most people. As you feel fit, you can increase the amount of time. Be mindful that overindulgence, even in exercise can be detrimental.

"Let your moderation be known unto all men...." Philippians 4:5

V

CAUTION: PLEASE CHECK WITH YOUR DOCTOR BEFORE BEGINNING AN EXERCISE PROGRAM.

ALSO CHECK WITH YOUR DOCTOR IF YOUR BODY FEELS TAXED IN ANY WAY REGARDLESS OF WHAT YOU HAVE BEEN ABLE TO DO IN THE PAST. BODIES AND ABILITIES CAN CHANGE. USE WISDOM!

"If any man lacks wisdom, ask of God who giveth liberally…."

James 1:5

V

CONCLUSION

"God giveth us richly all things to enjoy!"

I Timothy 6:17

As much as possible, spend time in nature. Let air into your dwelling. Go to where the air is clear. Practice inhalation and exhalation. Breathe deeply and slowly often throughout the day.

We were created in the image and the likeness of God. Therefore, let us depend on Him to give us the wisdom and knowledge to properly use what He has provided.

Let's take care of God's creation and do what we can to stick close to His plan.

PLAN! BALANCE! PRIORITIZE!

V

Do what is possible. God will do the rest.

"BELOVED, I WOULD THAT YOU WOULD PROSPER AND BE IN GOOD HEALTH, EVEN AS YOUR SOUL PROSPERS."

3 John 2

Enjoy every morning blessing!

Be blessed,

Veronica Gordon

RECIPES

By Veronica Gordon

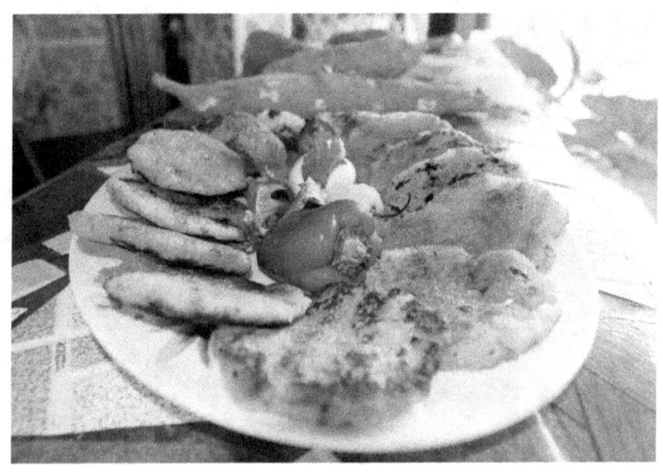

ENJOY A FEW NUTRITIOUS AND TASTY
CARRIBEAN DELIGHTS FROM VERONICA.

RECIPES

YUCCA TALL

Ingredients:

1Kilo grated raw yucca
3 cloves grater garlic
2 table spoon grater onion
2 table spoon chopped sweet pepper
2 table spoon chopped celery
2 table spoons chopped sweet cilantro
¼ tea spoon chopped aromatic pepper
½ tea spoon salt

Preparation:

1- In a deep bowl put the grated Yucca, then put all the other ingredients and mix well
2- Form the yucca tall.
3- Put some oil in the pan and put to heat and fry on medium heat.
4- Cover pan and keep watching until it gets a brown color and then flip it over and do the same processes until it gets brown on the other side.

You can have this for breakfast with scrambled eggs or for lunch.

Serves 6 people.

V

PATACONES DIP

(One of the Caribbean Specialties)

Ingredients for the patacones:

2 Green Plantains

1 cup of oil

Tip of salt

Preparation:

1- Peel the green plantains and cut it long way and then slice it in 4 pieces, you will have a total of 8 pieces for each plantain.
2- Pour the oil in the frying pan and put to heat.
3- When the pan is hot, put the plantain to fry on low to medium heat and wait till it gets soft.
4- Flip them over and wait until the other side is ready.
5- Take out the pieces and smash flat.
6- Fry them again with very high heat until they become crispy.
7- Add salt to state

V

Ingredients for the dip:

1 cup of cooked beans

1 table spoon chopped onion

1 table spoon chopped sweet pepper

1 table spoon chopped cilantro

2 cloves grated garlic

½ tea spoon aromatic pepper

¼ tea spoon curry

¼ cup water

Tip of black pepper

Salt to taste

Preparation:

Put all the ingredients in the blender and blend for 2 minutes

Put a spoon of oil into a hot pot and pour all the ingredients and cook for 10 minutes.

Serves 2 people

v

AREPA SESAME

<u>Ingredients:</u>

2 cups of wheat flour

1 cup of integral wheat flour

1 ¼ cups of water

Half teaspoon of salt

1 teaspoon of baking powder

4 tablespoons of coconut oil or any oil

2 tablespoons of sesame

1 frying pan

1 basin

<u>Preparation:</u>

Pour both flours. Mix all the dried ingredients in the basin. Add the oil (always keep mixing with your hands).

Pour the water gradually and keep mixing to form the dough.

V

Knead the dough for 3 minutes.

Separate manually the dough and form like little "tennis "balls (more or less)

Spread them out as a bread slice thickness on the table.

 Grease the pan, use medium heat, wait till hot and cook the arepas for 3 minutes with a cover.

Turn them over and let them cook for 3 additional minutes.

Turn over again for 2 minutes and ready to eat.

FRIED RIPEND PLANTAINS

Peel 2 plantains. Slice them not very thick.

Heat the pan (medium) and add ¼ of cup of coconut oil or other oil.

Fry until the plantains are golden and then turn them over and fry again.

Drain the excess of oil with kitchen paper on a plate.

V

MASHED BEANS

Ingredients:

1 cup of cooked beans

1 table spoon chopped onion

1 table spoon chopped sweet Pepper

1 table spoon chopped cilantro

2 cloves grated garlic

½ tea spoon aromatic pepper

¼ tea spoon curry

¼ cup water

Tip of black pepper

Salt to taste

Preparation:

Put all the ingredients in the blender and blend for 2 minutes

Put a spoon of oil into a hot pot and pour all the ingredients and cook for 10 minutes.

Serving size 2 people

With Appreciation

Many thanks to Veronica, her husband Delroy and their family for their hospitality during my stay in Puerto Viejo, Costa Rica. Their friendship, fellowship, wisdom and love are always appreciated. It was through my time with them that I was able to sample many of the delicious dishes featured in this book. To learn more about their story, please read "Veronica's Table," available on Amazon.com and Kindle.com

Other books by Ruth C. Chapman are also available on Amazon.com and Kindle.com

Feel free to Contact Ruth C. Chapman at
Rdestiny51@aol.com

Love and Blessings,

Ruth C. Chapman

V

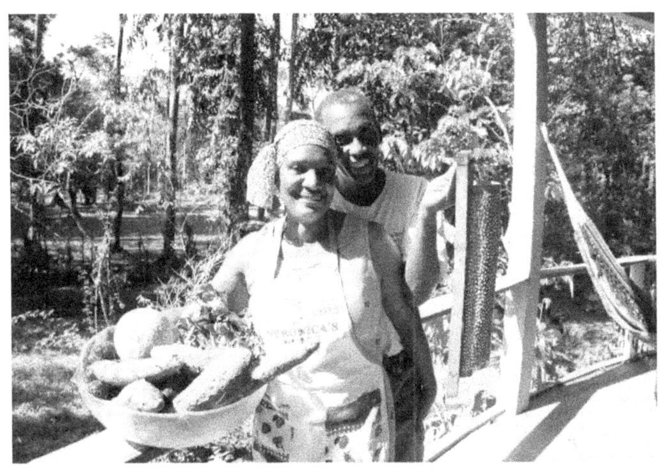

VERONICA AND HER HUSBAND DELROY

Visit Veronica and Delroy in Puerto Viejo, Costa Rica. They provide delectable vegan and vegetarian dishes, information on medicinal plants, wholistic healing, jungle tours and more.

Contact them at

veronicasplace@hotmail.com